CONTENTS

THE GLYCEMIA

TYPE II DIABETES, WHAT IT IS

PREVENT IT AND CURE
IT IN A NATURAL WAY

Dr. Gabriele Buracchi
Nutritionist and Psychologist

INTRODUCTION

According to CDC, 37.3 million people have diabetes, that's 11.3% of the US population.

In Italy, where I live, according to ISTAT 2015 data, 5.4% of Italians suffer from diabetes mellitus (both among males and females), for a total of over 3 million people. The areas in which the prevalence of diabetes is higher are the southern regions, in particular Calabria.

According to WHO, the number of people with diabetes

in the world, rose from 108 million in 1980 to 422 million in 2014.

These simple numbers say Diabetes is an increasing health problem-

Diabetes, or rather diabetes mellitus, depends on insulin. To be precise there may be:

- a reduced availability of insulin, therefore insufficient production for the body to function properly;

- poor sensitivity to the hormone by the target tissues, i.e. insulin is present, but the body is unable to make good use of it;

-the combination of these factors, i.e. insulin is low and does not work adequately.

The measurable consequence is hyperglycemia due to the aforementioned changes in insulin. Today they are distinguished:

TYPE 1 DIABETES

TYPE II DIABETES

GESTATIONAL DIABETES

Diabetes in the world population has increased in the

last 30-40 years to such an extent that there was talk of 108 million in 1980 against 422 million in 2014.

It is a metabolic disease due a decrease in the activity of insulin, a hormone produced by the beta cells of the islets of Langerhans in the pancreas.

The consequence is hyperglycemia, i.e. the excessive concentration of glucose in the blood.

Over time, it tends to be followed by complications of a vascular nature, such as:

-macroangiopathy (a particularly severe and early form of atherosclerosis).

Non-specific diabetes disorder.

-microangiopathy (disturbance of blood circulation within small arterial vessels, particularly in the retina, kidney and nerves).

Specific diabetes disorder.

CLASSIFICATION

The international classification of diabetes mellitus dates back to 1997 and identifies three main types:

TYPE 1 DIABETES MELLITUS.

It includes almost all forms of immune-mediated diabetes.

The underlying cause is therefore a malfunction of the immune system which recognizes the pancreatic *beta cells* of the insulin-producing islets of Langerhans as foreign, attacks and destroys them.

It is therefore an *autoimmune disease.*

TYPE II DIABETES MELLITUS.

It collects all forms due to a lack of insulin secretion by the pancreatic beta cells of the islets of Langerhans.

There is also resistance of the body's tissues to the action of insulin, a phenomenon called insulin resistance.

GESTATIONAL DIABETES.

Includes forms of diabetes secondary to pregnancy. Generally, it is a transient phenomenon.

I remind you that "*type 1 diabetes*" and "*type II diabetes*" also include forms associated with: viral infections (eg : rubella, cytomegalovirus), genetic syndromes (Down syndrome, Klinefelter syndrome, Turner syndrome, Friedreich ataxia, Laurence-Moon syndrome, myotonic dystrophy, Prader-Willi syndrome, Huntington 's chorea, etc.) but also hereditary genetic defects affecting the pancreatic beta cells of the islets of Langerhans known as MODY, i.e. *Maturity Onset Diabetes of the Young.*

Any form of diabetes mellitus may require insulin therapy and therefore the use of insulin by itself does not classify which form of diabetes is present.

This book mainly deals with type II diabetes, by far the most widespread, it being understood that the advice and dietary indications and natural therapies also apply to other forms, even if type 1 diabetes still requires the use of insulin and a medical check-up.

While not wanting and not being able to generalize, since each case is separate, I must say that in many years of professional practice the cases of type II diabetes that have followed my indications, have all resolved themselves better with a progressive abandonment of medications taken and a return of the glycemia and glycosylated hemoglobin values to normal values.

For this reason, before talking about diabetes, I anticipate a few simple notions on blood sugar and glycosylated hemoglobin.

GLYCEMIA

Glycemia comes from the ancient Greek: *glukýs*, "sweet" and *haîma*, "blood".

Glycemia indicates the concentration of glucose in the blood.

Glucose is an essential nutrient for all cells, which take it directly from the blood.

All the sugars that we ingest must be transformed into glucose to be used by the cells.

Glycemia regulation depends on specific hormones: hypoglycemic hormones lower the blood sugar level, like insulin, while hyperglycemic hormones, such as glucagon, raise it.

The balance between these hormones allows fasting values to be maintained in a range between 70 and 100 mg/dl in normal conditions.

Under normal conditions, after a meal, the pancreas increases the secretion of insulin to ensure that the glucose ingested with food is used by the cells.

In case of overweight or obesity, *"insulin resistance"* frequently develops, i.e. a condition characterized by a decreased ability of the cells of peripheral organs, in particular muscles, adipose tissue and liver, to respond to insulin.

In healthy subjects, with a regular life and a correct diet, blood glucose values usually fluctuate between 60 and 130 mg/dl during the day.

Fasting glycemic values can vary from 70 to 100 mg/dl.

Otherwise, if they are between **100 and 125 mg/dl**, we speak of impaired fasting glycemia, or *hyperglycemia*, a situation that should not be underestimated and which requires greater attention to lifestyle.

Values equal to, or greater than **126 mg/dl** are to be considered signs of a possible diabetes and further diagnostic investigations are required.

Below normal values **(less than 70 mg/dl)**, we speak of *hypoglycemia*.

GLYCOSYLATED OR GLYCATED HEMOGLOBIN

Hemoglobin becomes *glycosylated hemoglobin* if it is exposed to excessive concentrations of glucose in the blood, i.e. to high Glycemia.

Glycosylation is a modification of the structure of a protein.

It happens that a molecule of glucose binds to the hemoglobin present inside the red blood cells. For this reason, people with diabetes have higher levels of glycosylated hemoglobin (**HbA1c**) in red blood cells.

The modified hemoglobin is less effective at carrying oxygen in the blood.

It follows that the glycation of hemoglobin represents the major damage caused by diabetes.

This test is usually ordered only in people who are suspected of having diabetes.

This test is more useful than the standard blood glucose test -*Glycemia*- for diagnosing and monitoring diabetes due to the irreversibility of glycation.

The **glycosylated hemoglobin** inside the red blood cells

has the characteristic of remaining in circulation in the blood for about three or four months, i.e. for the average life span of a red blood cell.

In this way it allows you to have data regarding blood sugar over a long period, and not limited to a single moment.

SYMPTOMS OF TYPE II DIABETES

Type II diabetes is a chronic disease, that prevents the body from using insulin properly.

It is the result of increased insulin resistance and the pancreas not making enough insulin to handle blood sugar (glucose) levels.

Type II diabetes accounts for 90 to 95 percent of diabetes cases.

There are many symptoms of type II diabetes. It's important to know what they are because the condition can be prevented or delayed if caught early.

SIGNS OF TYPE II DIABETES

The symptoms of type II diabetes vary from person to person.

They can develop slowly over many years and may be so subtle that they are not noticed.

THE 3 P's OF DIABETES

Frequent Urination.

Excessive urination or **Polyuria**, is one of three.

The kidneys eventually cannot keep up with the extra glucose in the bloodstream.

Some of the glucose ends up in the urine and attracts more water.

This leads to more frequent urination.

Adults naturally produce 1 to 2 liters of urine per day. Polyuria is defined as more than 3 liters of urine per day[1].

Extreme Thirst.

Excessive thirst, or **Polydipsia**, is often the result of frequent urination.

The body pushes to replace lost fluids by making you feel thirsty.

Of course, everyone is thirsty sometimes.

Extreme thirst is unusual and persistent no matter how many times you drink.

Increased Hunger.

Excessive hunger is called **Polyphagia**.

With type 2 diabetes, the body has difficulty turning glucose into energy and this makes you hungry.

Eating introduces even more sugar that can't be processed and doesn't relieve hunger.

Blurred vision.

Diabetes increases the risk of several eye conditions [2], including: - diabetic retinopathy - cataracts - open-angle glaucoma,

Rising blood sugar due to diabetes can damage blood vessels [3], including those in the eye, leading to blurred vision.

Fatigue

Fatigue can be both mental and physical. There are many causes of tiredness.

It's a difficult symptom to research, but a 2016 study [4] concluded that people with type 2 diabetes may experience fatigue due to fluctuations between high and low glucose levels.

Slow-Healing Wounds

With type 2 diabetes, even minor cuts and scrapes can take longer to heal.

Foot injuries are common and easy to overlook. Slow-healing foot ulcers occur due to poor blood supply and damage to the nerves responsible for blood flow to the feet.

A 2020 study [5] demonstrated that diabetic foot ulcers

do not mobilize the immune cells necessary for proper inflammation and healing.

Tingling, numbness, and pain in hands and feet

High glucose can damage blood vessels that supply nutrients to nerves. When nerves don't get enough oxygen and nutrients, they can't function properly. This is called diabetic neuropathy and is more common in the extremities.

Unexplained Weight Loss

Insulin resistance causes glucose to build up in the bloodstream instead of being turned into energy.

This can cause the body to use up other sources of energy, such as muscle or fat tissue.

The weight could of course fluctuate slightly.

An unexplained loss of at least 5 percent of body weight warrants a doctor's visit.

Frequent Infections

In addition to nerve damage and a weakened immune system, poor blood circulation also increases the chance of developing an infection in people with diabetes.

Having more sugar in your blood and tissue allows infections to spread faster.

People with diabetes commonly develop infections [6] of the:

-ear, nose and throat

-kidney

-bladder

-feet

Areas of dark skin, such as the armpits or neck

Acanthosis nigricans is a skin condition that can be a symptom of diabetes. It appears as dark bands of skin that may have a velvety texture.

This is most common in body folds such as the armpits, neck and groin, but can occur elsewhere as well.

SYMPTOMS OF TYPE 2 DIABETES IN MEN

While the above symptoms can occur in anyone with type 2 diabetes, the following symptoms are specific to men:

-Men with diabetes have lower levels of testosterone, which one study [7] of 2016 tells us to be linked to a decrease in sexual desire.

-A 2017 research found that more than half of men with diabetes are affected by erectile dysfunction.

- Some men may experience retrograde ejaculation as a symptom of diabetes, according to research [8],[9]

- The lower testosterone levels seen in men with diabetes may also contribute to reduced muscle mass [10] .

SYMPTOMS OF DIABETES TYPE 2 DIABETES IN WOMEN

Type 2 diabetes can also present itself with symptoms specific to women, such as:

-Urinary tract infections are more common in women and are more common and severe in those with type 2 diabetes, according to research of 2015 [11].

- High glucose levels allow yeast organisms to grow more easily leading to a higher chance of infection [12].

Type II diabetes doesn't specifically make conception more difficult, but polycystic ovary syndrome (PCOS) does.

The development of PCOS has been linked to insulin resistance, and PCOS has been shown to increase the risk of type 2 diabetes, according to the CDC [13].

ARE THERE SYMPTOMS OF PREDIABETES 2?

Prediabetes is a health condition in which your blood sugar is higher than it should be, but isn't high enough to allow a diagnose of type 2 diabetes.

Usually, there are no symptoms of prediabetes, but there are steps you can take to avoid developing it [14].

-losing excess weight and maintaining a moderate weight

-exercising as often as possible

-adapting your diet, focusing on a nutrient-rich and balanced meal plan

-drinking water instead of low-nutrient beverages such as sugary drinks, anyway dangerous for health.

Having prediabetes does not mean you will definitely develop diabetes, although it is important to make dietary and lifestyle changes to prevent the condition from progressing.

It is estimated that between 15% and 30% of people [15] with prediabetes will develop diabetes within the next 3-5 years if no lifestyle changes are made.

If this happens, the consequences are those of diabetes.

HOW TO REDUCE THE RISK

A large multi-center research study called *Diabetes Prevention Program* looked at how lifestyle changes can help prevent diabetes.

What they found should give people at risk for diabetes much hope.

With modest weight loss and exercise, study participants reduced their risk of developing diabetes by 58% over 3 years [16].

Therefore, making dietary and lifestyle changes can be especially helpful for those with prediabetes and can help support blood sugar control and overall health.

CAUSES OF TYPE II DIABETES

There is not a single cause, but in fact there can be a combination of factors leading to type II diabetes.

Let's look at certain factors associated with type II diabetes below.

Genetics and Family History

Genetics appear to play a significant role in a person's risk of developing type II diabetes.

In fact, the link between type II diabetes and family history is stronger than the link between type 1 diabetes and family history, according to *American Diabetes Association* [17].

Insulin Resistance

The body uses a hormone called insulin to help glucose in the bloodstream get into cells, so it can be used for energy, but a condition called insulin resistance can develop when cells in muscle, fat, and of the liver do not respond well to the action of insulin.

This makes it more difficult for glucose to enter cells.

As a result, too much remains in the bloodstream.

The pancreas is forced to increase secretion by producing more and more insulin, but it becomes progressively harder to keep up and blood sugar levels remain elevated.

This prepares you for developing prediabetes or type II diabetes.

Visceral fat

A certain type of fat, called visceral fat, can increase the risk of type II diabetes.

It is the fat that surrounds [18] internal organs, such as the liver and intestines, deep within the trunk.

While visceral fat is only about 10% of total body fat, it has the highest associated risk of metabolic problems, such as insulin resistance.

In fact, research suggests that people with larger waistlines, who therefore may have more of this belly fat, are at higher risk for type 2 diabetes [19].

Sedentary Lifestyle

Sitting for long periods of time can increase the risk of developing type II diabetes.

It has been shown [20] that regular physical activity can

help to better control blood glucose levels.

Certain medications

It is possible that certain medications for another medical condition may predispose the subject to developing type II diabetes.

For example, **corticosteroids** [21] such as *prednisone*, are often used to treat inflammation, but are also associated with the risk of developing diabetes.

High doses of *statins*, used to treat high cholesterol, can also increase the risk.

Other medications that have been linked to an increased risk of developing diabetes in some cases include:

-beta-blockers

-second generation antipsychotic drugs

-thiazide diuretics

Other medications can also raise blood sugar levels, so it may be worth talking about with a doctor if you start taking a new drug, especially if you have other risk factors for type II diabetes. It is important to note that medications should not be stopped without consulting a doctor.

Certain medical conditions

If the subject has prediabetes, his blood sugar levels are

high but not high enough for a diagnosis of diabetes. Usually it is enough to eat the right foods and practice a little physical activity to return to normal values. Obviously, if the habits remain the same, the probability of reaching full-blown diabetes is high. Other conditions that may increase your risk of developing type II diabetes include:

-high blood pressure

-heart disease

-a history of stroke

-polycystic ovary syndrome (PCOS)

-having low HDL cholesterol and high triglyceride levels.

DOES SUGAR CAUSE DIABETES?

Some people believe that consuming sugar alone, can cause type II diabetes to develop.

However, this is only true under certain conditions only.

According to a 2015 study [22] published in the *Journal of Diabetes Investigation*, drinking lots of sodas and sugary drinks is definitely associated with a higher risk of type II diabetes, but natural sugars, like those in fresh fruit, don't.

Even this large Chinese study [23] found that a greater consumption of fresh fruit was associated with a significantly lower risk of diabetes and, among diabetic individuals, with lower risks of death and development of major vascular complications.

Whether someone will develop diabetes depends on many other factors, such as the ones mentioned above.

Eating a nutrient-rich diet and getting regular physical activity will improve your health on many fronts, including reducing your likelihood of developing type II diabetes.

Other risk factors, in addition to familiarity, concern age.

While type II diabetes can develop at any age, it is also true that people over the age of 45 are at the greatest risk of type II diabetes.

There are differences based on race/ethnicity.

In the United States, type II diabetes is more common among African Americans, although this is likely due to a combination of factors, including access and inequalities in health care.

In addition to this, people who develop gestational diabetes during pregnancy are more likely to develop type II diabetes later in life.

Research [24] estimates that between 15 and 70 percent of people with gestational diabetes are more likely to develop diabetes.

RATIO BETWEEN VITAMIN D AND DIABETES

A recent study [25] published by the *European Journal of Endocrinology* set out to determine whether consistent vitamin D3 supplementation could improve insulin sensitivity in patients newly diagnosed with type II diabetes or at high risk of developing the disease.

Comprised of 96 randomized patients, the double-blind, placebo-controlled study administered patients 5,000 international units (IU) per day for 6 months.

"In individuals at high risk for diabetes or with newly diagnosed type II diabetes, vitamin D supplementation for 6 months significantly increased peripheral insulin sensitivity and beta-cell function, suggesting it may slow metabolic deterioration in this population" was the result.

Some previous studies had yielded modest results, but the researchers suggest that previous studies may have failed to demonstrate the benefits of vitamin D supplementation due to variables including ethnicity, glucose tolerance, and vitamin D dosage and duration during the study.

Diabetes care experts validate a true link between diabetes and vitamin D.

But what is the link between vitamin D and diabetes?

Low vitamin D levels are a prevalent problem in people with and without diabetes worldwide. Research has repeatedly found a clear association between low vitamin D levels in patients with insulin resistance and a high risk of developing type II diabetes, as shown in a 2011 Canadian study [26].

This study appears to demonstrate that with supplementation before diagnosis, or soon after, the body retains the ability to respond better at the cellular level to insulin, which counteracts the hallmark of type II diabetes: insulin resistance.

The other thing that seems to help is allowing the insulin-producing beta cells in the pancreas to remain healthy and functional.

Beta cells play a central role in insulin secretion. Gradual beta-cell dysfunction is the main culprit of type II diabetes for about 60% of people diagnosed with it, according to a 2016 study [27].

Vitamin D can positively impact insulin secretion in several ways, we are told by a research conducted by the

National Institute of health [28].

Vitamin D enters the beta cell and interacts with different types of receptors, which bind to each other and essentially activate the insulin gene, increasing insulin synthesis.

Vitamin D is also thought to help beta cells survive in a person with diabetes

- whose body is otherwise trying to gradually destroy those cells - by interfering with the effects of cytokines, which are produced by the immune system.

Vitamin D also plays a vital role in regulating the body's use of calcium.

And calcium actually plays a small but vital role in insulin secretion.

If too little vitamin D impairs the body's ability to manage calcium levels, it inevitably impairs the body's ability to produce insulin.

Through the same receptors associated with vitamin D's impact on insulin secretion, vitamin D stimulates receptors that affect insulin sensitivity.

Through a complicated physiological process, interacting with and binding to these receptors actually increases the total number of insulin receptors present in the body.

Vitamin D is also thought to improve insulin sensitivity

by activating other receptors that help regulate fatty acid metabolism in muscle and body fat.

The relationship of vitamin D with calcium and insulin secretion is related to the fact that the presence of calcium is essential for the insulin response of muscle and fat, allowing for the uptake of insulin and glucose.

Without calcium, this cannot happen.

And without vitamin D, there's no calcium.

GETTING TO KNOW CARBOHYDRATES TO USE THEM AT THE BEST

As it appears clear from what has been said in the text, in principle and with a few exceptions, what gives rise to type II diabetes is excess blood sugar due to excess carbohydrates.

But are all carbohydrates created equal?

Do sugar or zucchini have the same effect?

Let's start by understanding what is gathered under this broad definition of Carbohydrates. Carbohydrates, Proteins and Fats are collectively called MACRONUTRIENTS.

Carbohydrates, those that have the main effect on blood sugar and therefore insulin, are a very diverse category.

The most wrong thing that can be done in the field of food is to generalize, to believe that there are damned foods and others to be consumed without limits.

The truth, and common sense, lie somewhere in between these extremes.

This logically also applies to carbohydrates or carbon hydrates, also known as glycides (*from the Greek gluco or glico , i.e. sweet*) or sugars.

What we can immediately say is that carbohydrates are not all "*good*", nor all "*bad*".

Some types of Carbohydrates are healthy and useful for health, we could say absolutely indispensable, while others, if eaten frequently and in large quantities, in addition to making you fat, increase the risk of suffering from diabetes and cardiovascular system diseases, but not only this.

Still others, such as alcohol and sodas, are to be avoided in any dose, not only for the sugar they bring, but also for their content in toxic substances.

If it is certainly true that refined, easily digestible carbohydrates, such as those contained in white bread, white rice, puff pastry, sugary drinks, alcohol - *yes, alcohol is also a sugar, suffice it to say that a glass of red wine contains about 70 Kcal* - and in other preserved foods, they can make you fat, or cause blood sugar to rise rapidly, it is equally true that whole grains are already better and that legumes, fruit, vegetables have an opposite effect, allowing those who consume to stay healthy.

What are carbohydrates for?

We must never forget that our body uses Carbohydrates to synthesize **Glucose**, that is the *"petrol"* that allows us to live and without which our life would not be possible. The problem is, if anything, the speed with which glucose is produced and its quantity, two fundamental factors which, however, are under the direct control of our food choices.

Carbohydrates are found in these foods:

-fruit
-vegetables
-bread, cereals and cereal-based products
-milk and dairy products
-sugar itself and foods with added sugar (for example cakes, biscuits and sweetened drinks)
-alcohol
Foods that we can consider healthy and useful to our life and health are:
- those rich in dietary fiber such as whole grains and those with no added sugar
- fruit and vegetables (with some attention)

THE FIRST DISTINCTION TO MAKE.

This is a first fundamental distinction that makes us understand how those foods rich in simple carbohydrates, such as soft drinks, alcohol, all junk food with added sugars should be eliminated, while refined products such as bread, pasta, non-wholemeal rice should in any case be to be viewed with suspicion and certainly to be used moderately and occasionally.

Moreover, they only bring calories and no other nutrients to the diet. Carbohydrates, therefore, once this distinction has been made, are a fundamental part of a healthy diet, because they give the body the petrol it needs for physical activity and for the correct functioning of the organs. The best sources of carbohydrates are therefore fruit, vegetables, legumes and whole cereals, which also provide essential vitamins, minerals and fibres, as well as absolutely essential antioxidants which cannot be found elsewhere.

WHAT ARE CARBOHYDRATES

They are nutrients found in many different foods in various forms. The most widespread and abundant in nature are: - sugars - fibers - starches

The fundamental element of all carbohydrates is a

molecule of glucose, a combination of carbon, hydrogen and oxygen.

Starches and fibers are nothing more than more or less long chains of glucose molecules: the chains can also contain hundreds of sugar molecules and be straight or extremely branched.

DIVIDED INTO 2 GROUPS.

In the past, carbohydrates were divided into two groups:
1) **Simple**, including sugars such as fructose (fruit sugar), dextrose or glucose (wheat or grape sugars) and sucrose (table sugar).
2) **Complexes**, including molecules consisting of more than three glucose molecules.

It used to be simplistically thought that complex carbohydrates were better, although it turns out that the picture is not as simple as previously thought.

Much of the credit for this comes from the studies on the **Glycemic Index and the Glycemic Load**, which are discussed in the following chapters.

The digestive system treats all Carbohydrates in more or less the same way: it breaks them down or tries to break them down into the glucose molecules that make them up, or into the molecules of other simple sugars, then converting them into glucose, because the body's cells are programmed to use Glucose as a universal energy source.

SIMPLE CARBOHYDRATES.

They include sugars that occur naturally in fruits, vegetables, milk and dairy products, but also sugars added during food storage and preparation.

In general, foods with added sugars contain fewer nutrients than other foods.

One way to avoid ingesting added sugars is to read the ingredients list on food labels.

Added sugars are typically listed as:

-Brown sugar

-Corn syrup

-Dextrose

-Fructose

-Fruit juice concentrate

-Glucose

-High fructose corn syrup

-Honey

-Invert sugar

-Lactose

-Maltose

- Malt Syrup

- Molasses

- Sugar

- Sucrose

- Syrup

The higher the ingredient is on the ingredients list, the higher the added sugar content of the food.

We can then take other measures to reduce the consumption of added sugars:

-Drink water instead of sweetened carbonated drinks, which also contain other substances that are very harmful to health

-Drink real fruit juice and not packaged juices, moreover obtained from fruit waste.

-Eat some fresh fruit instead of dessert and avoid desserts with added sugar

-If you like breakfast cereals, choose breakfast cereals with no added sugar

It is probably known that sugars and starches are a key factor in the formation of caries, but it is still useful to remember this, especially with regard to children. To prevent cavities, it is therefore important to reduce or eliminate simple sugars, as well as brushing and flossing your teeth.

COMPLEX CARBOHYDRATES: STARCHES AND DIETARY FIBERS.

Starches must be modified through digestion before the

body can use them as a source of glucose.

They are the main energy reserve of plants, where it is mainly concentrated in tubers, such as potatoes and tapioca, and in seeds, such as rice, corn and wheat.

Starch in its native state comes in the form of granules, with variable

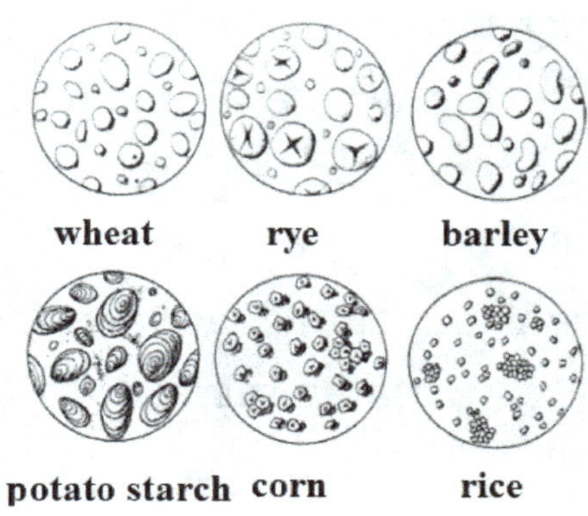

Various forms of starches

shapes and sizes depending on the plants from which it derives.

From a chemical point of view, starch is a polysaccharide made up of two glucose polymers:

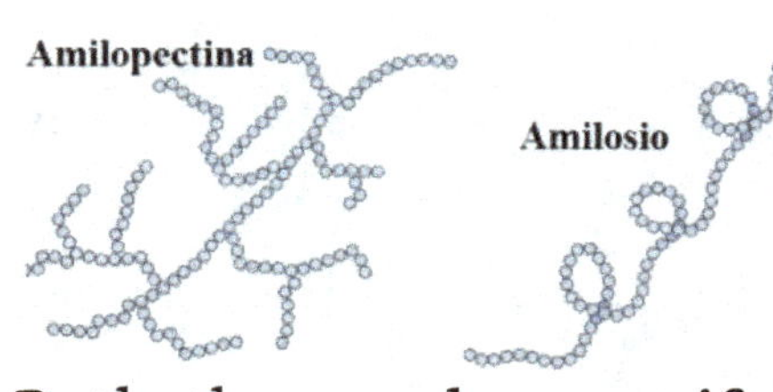

- **a linear one, called Amylose (20%)**

- **a branched one, called Amylopectin (80%)**

Both these polymers, if treated with diluted acids or with enzymes, break down further, down to single units of glucose.

These reactions take place in our body through the work of salivary (ptyaline), pancreatic (amylase) and intestinal (dextrinase , maltase) enzymes , with the contribution of gastric acidity which favors the breaking of raw or resistant granules.

Fibers

Dietary fibers are indicated on food labels as either soluble or insoluble.

Soluble fiber is found in these foods:

- oatmeal

- bran

- nuts and seeds

-in most types of fruit (for example, strawberries, blueberries, pears and apples)

- beans and dried legumes

Insoluble fiber, on the other hand , can be found in these foods:

- whole wheat bread

- barley

- brown rice

- couscous

- bulgur or whole wheat cereals

- bran

- seeds,

- most vegetables

- fruit

But what's the best type of fiber?

Both are, since each has important health benefits, so

getting all of these foods into your diet is essential to get enough of both types of fiber.

It will obviously be easier to get the other nutrients by choosing foods that are high in fiber. -Soluble fibers bind to fats in the intestines and transport them away in the form of waste substances.

In this way they reduce **bad cholesterol (LDL)**; they also serve to regulate the body's use of sugars, because they keep the hunger stimulus and blood sugar under control. -Insoluble fibers facilitate intestinal transit, because they promote regularity and help prevent constipation.

THREE FUNDAMENTAL PARAMETERS

Whether you suffer from diabetes or you don't want to run the risk of encountering it, there are three fundamental parameters to know, very simple concepts, within anyone's reach, which can make a fundamental difference.

These are the Glycemic Index GI, the Glycemic Load GL and the Insulin Index II.

Since, as we have said, type II diabetes is basically based on dietary errors that cause strong fluctuations in blood sugar, let's try to understand what causes these fluctuations and what instead protects us from them.

Let's see how we can predict this in a very simple way, knowledge that allows us to be able to better evaluate and organize our diet.

Further on you will find the link to the international glycemic index tables, but it is very simple to find the glycemic indexes of various foods and their available carbohydrates on the Internet.

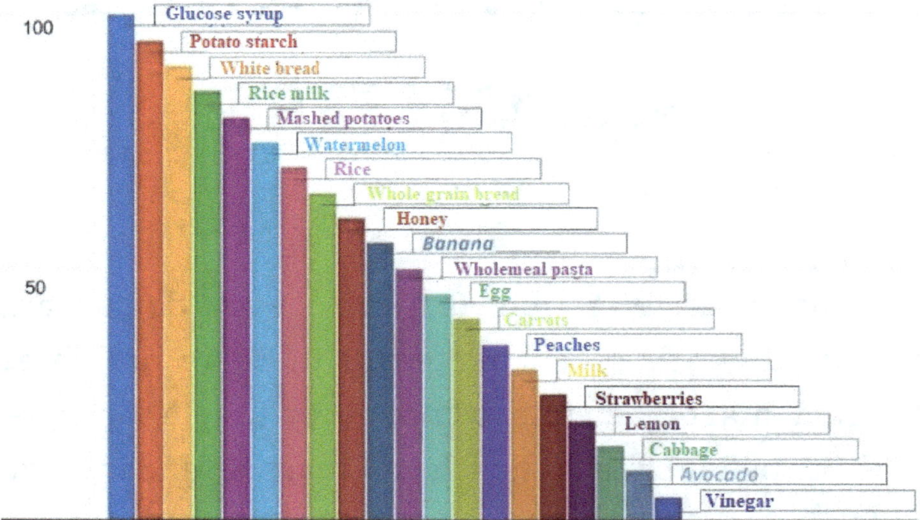

THE GLYCEMIC INDEX

Why isn't it indifferent to the type of carbohydrate we eat?

Why isn't it the same thing to eat, for example, 100 grams of salad and 100 grams of pasta?

And why is the former definitely a much better source of carbohydrates than the latter?

Apart from the enormous importance of the vitamins, antioxidants, mineral salts and fibers that salad (taken here for example from vegetables) contains and which pasta contains only insignificantly, a fundamental difference is constituted by the different speed with which these two foods cause blood sugar to rise, consequently causing a different production of insulin.

All this depends on a very important factor, the Glycemic Index, developed in the early 80s but unfortunately still ignored or misunderstood even by many *experts* in the sector.

UNDERSTANDING WHAT THE GLYCEMIC INDEX (GI) IS

Let's consider a cup of sugar, a rice cake, some bread,

some cherries, some zucchini, and finally a sheet of paper - perhaps the one on which your trusted nutritionist has wrote the diet - in any case we took a CARBOHYDRATE - or glycide, which we can also more confidently call sugar. In fact, sugars are not only those foods that appear sweet to the taste.

VARIETY OF CARBOHIDRATES IN NATURE.

There are many types of carbohydrates, or sugars, in nature. Some, such as cellulose, pectins, hemicelluloses, as well as a wide range of gums and mucilages of various origins, are classified as fibers, i.e. they are not digestible and therefore cannot be used for energy purposes by our body.

They are only "*ballast*", but precious ballast for other functions they perform.

Yet cellulose, used to make paper, is made up of glucose molecules just like spaghetti or bread or rice.

Only that the type of chemical bond with which these glucose molecules are linked together makes them unusable for us.

It's a shame, because while spaghetti also contains other substances in a small percentage, cellulose only contains glucose.

The fact is that our digestive system is not able to

separate the bonds that unite these glucose molecules, something that ruminants and herbivores in general do very well.

For them, cellulose is a good food that allows them to live.

SIMPLE AND COMPLEX CARBOHYDRATES.

The carbohydrates assimilable to us are classified, from a nutritional point of view, as "simple" or as "complex".

Among the complex ones, in addition to fibers, we remember starch, made up of linear (amylose) and branched (amylopectin) in variable proportions.

Simple carbohydrates, commonly called sugars, include monosaccharides such as glucose, the most common organic compound in nature - and fructose, - fruit sugar, present in many fruits and in some types of honey - , and disaccharides, such as sucrose – the common cooking sugar extracted from beets or sugar cane -, maltose – made up of two glucose molecules joined together through α bonds (1 $\rightarrow$ 4) and which in nature is found in discrete quantities only in sprouted seeds - and lactose - milk sugar -

Although they are already naturally present in primary foods, sugars in refined form are used as such (sucrose) or incorporated into foods and drinks to increase their pleasantness, thanks to their sweet taste. Until recently, it was believed that the speed of absorption of carbohydrates depended on their greater or lesser complexity.

It seemed logical to assume that pasta, mainly composed of long glucose molecules joined together, required much more time to enter the circulation than, for example, fructose, the sugar extracted from fruit, which is a simple sugar.

HOW WE ASSIMILATE CARBOHYDRATES

Checking the increase in blood sugar after the ingestion of a food, however, we realized that the body follows different logics from those of some theories, logics that determine greater or lesser capacity to make us fat, but not only this.

In fact, the body assimilates carbohydrates on the basis of their **Glycemic Index (GI)**, which represents the speed with which blood sugar (i.e. glycemia) increases after consuming **50 grams** of the carbohydrate in question.

Speed is expressed as a percentage by taking glucose (50 g.) as a reference point, i.e. by attributing it a value of 100.

This happens because the human body can only use the ingested sugars, of any type, by transforming them all into glucose.

Sometimes, GI tables are found that take bread as a base 100.

In this case, just multiply the value by 0.73 to obtain the value on the glucose scale.

WHAT DO THE DIFFERENT RATES OF ASSIMILATION MEAN.

If the food being examined has a glycemic index of 50, this means that the food being examined raises blood sugar with a speed equal to half that of glucose, while if it is 25, the speed will be equal to a quarter. and so on.

By going to see the GI of various foods, we thus discover some facts that were not even conceivable just a few years ago.

The same quantity of spaghetti, for example, a food considered a complex carbohydrate, can have a glycemic index ranging from about 35 to over 60 - it must always be remembered that glucose is worth 100 - depending on whether it is undercooked or overcooked spaghetti.

Fructose, a simple sugar which, among other things, has the same calories by weight as cooking sugar, has a GI of 23, while the same cooking sugar, sucrose, in fact, has a GI of 68 , therefore not very different from that of well-cooked pasta.

The different consequences of ingesting high GI or low

GI carbohydrates, regardless of whether they are simple carbohydrates or complex carbohydrates, can be seen in the graph.

Why does this happen? It's pretty simple.

Because every time blood sugar rises quickly, the pancreas will quickly release a proportional dose of insulin, the assimilation and accumulation hormone, into the circulation.

EFFECTS OF HIGH AND LOW GI. HIGH

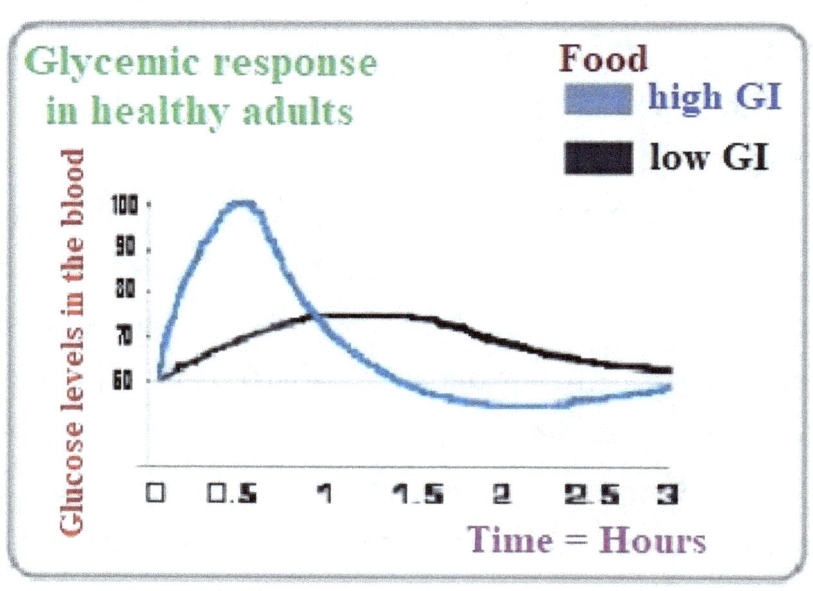

Glycemic response in healthy adults

High GI foods – as can be clearly seen by looking at the graph – will cause blood sugar to rise very quickly but, due to the effect of the insulin produced, it will quickly drop below the average level, leading to a situation of hypoglycemia.

The energy taken up very quickly will be spent by the body only in part.

When we "*fill up*" with high GI carbohydrates, we cause an excessive increase in glucose - our fuel - in the blood.

Since the body is not able to tolerate hyperglycemia that much, insulin readily produced by the pancreas (under normal conditions) stores glucose in the form of fat; as a result, there will be a situation of hypoglycemia and therefore hunger, obviously for carbohydrates.

GETTING FAT AND HUNGRY?

Basically we will end up gaining weight and being hungry at the same time. The worst solution Unlike what happens with foods with a high GI, foods with a low glycemic index, by slowly releasing glucose into the circulation, will on the contrary allow energy to be made available gradually, giving the body time to consume it all without accumulating a more or less abundant part as fat.

A key side effect is not to stress the pancreas to produce a surplus of insulin.

The practical consequences of what we have said are that the more we eat foods with a high GI, the easier it will be to gain weight, but immediately before this we will have created strong fluctuations in blood sugar.

So first of all we have to keep under control products such as sweets -obviously- but also bread, pasta, potatoes and in particular french fries but also carbonated drinks, rich in sugar and alcohol. All of these foods, including sodas, are basically all sugars and very fast sugars.

The main responsible for our fattening.

We always remember that wholemeal products have a slightly lower GI than refined equivalents, but also that a low GI product like most vegetables, if combined with a high GI product, such as pasta, reduces the risk of gaining weight.

Even proteins, when associated with carbohydrates, slow down their GI Choosing foods based on the glycemic index is essential!

Fats, finally, do not affect the GI in the slightest .

On the contrary, within certain limits, fats are needed in order not to gain weight.

Therefore, instead of a plate of spaghetti without anything else, a plate of spaghetti is better, however much smaller than we are used to eating, seasoned with a little oil, with lots of vegetables and always associated with a second course.

In fact, the basis of our diet should be made up of fruit and vegetables with the right amount of protein and vegetable fats such as olive oil.

Unfortunately in western countries the idea has prevailed, probably driven by interested advertisements, that the famous Mediterranean diet consists of a nice plate of pasta or potatoes or bread.

Nothing more false and dangerous. The basic foods of the Mediterranean diet are fruit, vegetables, legumes, olive oil but also fish or white meat.

And if you prefer a vegetarian diet, soy and lupine provide sufficient proteins.

LOSE WEIGHT, BUT SLOWLY.

Here's the best way not to gain weight again. It is therefore essential to lose weight only if really necessary, but above all in a slow and progressive way.

This will make it possible not to gain weight again at the end of the slimming diets, but also to avoid stretch marks and other skin blemishes that are always created in rapid slimming. The dangers of fast weight loss diets. Losing weight with slimming diets that make you lose weight quickly is not only wrong but downright dangerous. From what has been said on the GI, Glycemic Index, consequences arise that cannot be overlooked if you really want to lose weight by avoiding the well-known Jo-Jo effect, or *cyclical weight swing syndrome*, as it is called in scientific jargon.

Unlike what was thought in the past – but unfortunately many continue to believe – the importance of total calories in a diet is significantly reduced.

It is not the same to assume, for example, 300 kilocalories from a low GI food such as vegetables or from a high GI food such as a dessert, but also from bread and pasta.

The value of the difference between simple and complex carbohydrates is also greatly reduced, given that the GI of a complex carbohydrate such as pasta, especially if well cooked, is very close to that of a simple carbohydrate such as table sugar -sucrose- and is much higher than that of fructose, a simple sugar extracted from fruit.

If the GI of pasta varies according to the greater or lesser cooking, so also a ripe fruit has a higher GI than an unripe fruit.

Even the GI of bread varies according to the method of production and cooking.

The Glycemic Index is also influenced by interactions with fats and proteins.

For a balanced and at the same time pleasant diet, whether you want to lose weight or want to maintain your weight, it is decidedly preferable to associate a carbohydrate-based meal – such as the classic pasta dish – with protein foods such as meat or fish or legumes, adding a certain amount of vegetable fats – olive oil – as the presence of these two macronutrients slows down the speed of intestinal absorption.

WHAT MUST NEVER BE MISSING.

Vegetables must not be missing, which with their fibers will help to modulate, reducing it, the increase in blood sugar induced by pasta.

It is therefore nutritionally more indicated to eat a plate of pasta with tomato sauce with a can of tuna rather than eating the same amount of pasta without seasonings.

Of course it is much more correct to eat a smaller amount of pasta, since we have proteins and a large dose of vegetables at our disposal.

But, it should be pointed out, pasta that is now passed off as a traditional food, has nothing to do with the Mediterranean diet and is indeed a bad food.

Adding a spoonful of olive oil, in addition to slowing down the subsequent onset of hunger, also decreases the Glycemic Index of the meal taken as a whole.

GLYCEMIC LOAD

What does the **Glycemic Load (GL)** tell us more than the Glycemic Index (GI) ?

The effects that foods have on the body, in particular foods that act on blood sugar, depend, as already mentioned, on their Glycemic Index, but also on the ingested quantities of that food.

IMPORTANCE OF AVAILABLE CARBOHYDRATES.

This means taking into account the Glycemic Load (GL), a parameter which, in addition to the Glycemic Index (GI), also depends on the quantity of Available Carbohydrates (AC) in a food.

It is intuitive that it is not the same thing, from the point of view of glycemia, to eat 50g of pasta or to eat 100, even if it is the same pasta and therefore with the same GI.

As we said when speaking of the GI, we consider sugar (understood as sucrose), rice cakes, bread, cherries, courgettes and, finally, the sheet of paper on which your nutritionist has written your diet.

To calculate the **Glycemic Load**, I apply the following formula.

The formula for calculating the glycemic load is $= \dfrac{GI \times AC}{100} = GL$

Looking at the table, it becomes clear why a diet that does not cause blood sugar to rise much, becomes more sustainable if rich in fruit and vegetables.

Practical examples.

Carbohydrate	Glycemic Index	Available Carbohydrates %	Glycemic Load
Sugar (sucrose)	68	100	6800/100 = 68
Rice crackers	85	80	6800/100 = 68
White bread	70	56	3920/100 = 39,2
Cherries	22	11,7	257,4/100 = 2,5
Courgettes	15	2,3	34,5/100 = 0,3
Sheet of paper	0	0	0

As it is evident from the table, in fact, eating table sugar (sucrose) or the same dose of rice crackers will have the same effect on our Glycenia, and therefore on our body. And to think that there are people who consume rice crackers believing that it is a slimming product!!!

If instead we look at the data of cherries, representative of fruit, or courgettes, representative of vegetables, we realize that their Glycemic Load is so low as to be practically insignificant.

This is why we can safely eat large doses of fruit and almost unlimited doses of vegetables, without consequences on blood sugar, i.e. without gaining weight and without causing dangerous fluctuations in blood sugar.

Of course, even among fruits and vegetables there are some limited exceptions, but they are still exceptions, and in any case very relative, as in the case of bananas or carrots.

Our sheet of paper, placed there to represent nutritionally inert carbohydrates , i.e. fibers, gives a glycemic load of 0.

But despite this, it is strongly advised not to eat paper!!

International index and glycemic load tables here, [29].

INSULIN INDEX

The **Insulin Index** is, perhaps, less known than other parameters, but it is of undoubted importance.

Given the importance that insulin production has on our health and well-being, in more recent times , another parameter called the **Insulin Index (II)** has been established.

Insulin Index measures the production of insulin in the body in response to the ingestion of any food, therefore independently of blood sugar (Glycemia).

In fact, the **Insulin Index** measures the effect of a food exclusively and directly on insulinemia , allowing a more precise assessment of the insulin response exclusively with the same caloric value of all foods.

This index, therefore, makes it possible to evaluate whether any food, not necessarily a carbohydrate, is capable of causing a low, moderate or high insulin response.

Indeed, the impact of macronutrients on insulinemia is 90-100% for Carbohydrates, 50% for Proteins and 10% for Fats, and this confirms that it is not only Carbohydrates that affect insulin production, but also

Proteins in a moderate way, and Fats in a very mild way, which the Glycemic Index does not consider.

It thus turns out that some foods manage to stimulate **insulin** in a disproportionate way with respect to their Glycemic Index and Load, and that the mixed meal in any case determines a production of the hormone much higher than its carbohydrate content, and therefore still at the Glycemic Index and Glycemic Load.

Many investigations have shown that the *insulinogenic effect* of dairy products is three to six times higher than their corresponding glycemic index.

It has also been understood that it is not the lipids, i.e. the fats, of the milk that cause such a marked difference between the glycemic index and the insulin index, as both whole and skimmed milk do not present significant differences in their values.

On the other hand, it is in particular the fraction of whey proteins that gives milk the greatest insulinotropic properties, contrary to what happens with meat.

A study that evaluated 38 types of foods, showed that meat and fish have a low Glycemic Index, but a medium Insulin Index, while yogurt has a medium Glycemic Index and a very high Insulin Index.

Interesting is the case of the artificial sweetener **Acesulfame K** which, being devoid of caloric intake, obviously does not affect blood sugar but nevertheless stimulates insulin in a dose-response manner with levels similar to the same amount of glucose. Yet another reason to avoid this and all other artificial sweeteners.

In the case of the classic Italian breakfast consisting of croissant and cappuccino, there is a hyperinsulinizing and hypoglycaemic effect due to insulin, abundantly stimulated in a synergistic way by refined flour, sugar and hydrogenated fats contained in the croissant, together with milk and sugar of the cappuccino.

FOOD TIPS TO FIGHT AND PREVENT TYPE II DIABETES

If it is certain that all low-calorie diets, if followed, lead to a reduction in body weight, it is equally certain that there are substantial differences in the type of loss recorded in according to the diet undertaken.

But keep in mind that weight loss is only an indicator of the condition of blood sugar.

In fact, one cannot speak of health benefits and maintenance of the results obtained over time in the case of weight loss due to dehydration that is obtained with ketogenic diets, or in weight reduction obtained by self-cannibalization of muscles and internal organ structures as happens with low protein diets.

The only diets that have beneficial and lasting effects are those that only lead to the loss of excess accumulated body fat.

But if you lose weight this way, that's just an indication that your blood sugar no longer rises so high that new fat accumulates.

On the contrary! We reversed the process.

Precisely on this aspect the **Zone diet** has proven to be superior to all other more or less bizarre and imaginative diets, in consuming fat more quickly [30],[31],[32],[33] and for this reason I would recommend it after having followed hundreds of people with type II diabetes over the years.

Studies have shown that if a person has an initial elevated insulin response resulting from the glucose stimulus, the Zone Diet has superior weight loss efficacy [34],[35].

A study published in the New England Journal of Medicine points out that a diet with a composition similar to the Zone is better than others in maintaining the weight loss achieved[36].

This fact is probably caused by an increase in perceived satiety induced by the Zone diet compared to other diets [37],[38].

DIABETES AND ZONE, THE IMPORTANCE.

These characteristics of the Zone are of primary importance in all types of diabetes, from type 1 diabetes which usually has an acute onset and which in any case affects about 5/10% of people with diabetes and generally arises in childhood or in adolescence.

In type 1 diabetes, the pancreas does not produce insulin

due to the destruction of the beta cells that produce this hormone: it is therefore necessary that it be injected every day and for life.

A balanced diet like the Zone, together with the right physical exercise, does not eliminate the need for insulin injections, but it can reduce their quantity, with many beneficial effects.

Then there is the type II diabetes, which manifest itselves more slowly and often in a less evident way.

There are cases of high Glycemia occuring without symptoms even for long periods of time. There are also clinical situations in which Glycemia does not exceed the levels established for the definition of diabetes, but which, in any case, do not constitute a normal condition .

In these cases we speak of **Impaired Fasting Glycemia (IFG)** when the fasting blood glucose values are between 100 and 125 mg/dl and Impaired Glucose Tolerance (IGT) when the blood glucose two hours after the glucose load is between 140 and 200 mg/dl.

This is the so-called "pre-diabetes" we have spoken about, which indicates a high risk of developing diabetic disease.

It is often associated with overweight, dyslipidemia and/ or hypertension and is accompanied by an increased risk of cardiovascular events.

Finally, we recall gestational diabetes, defined as when a high level of circulating glucose is measured for the first time during pregnancy.

This condition occurs in about 4% of pregnancies.

The first publication confirming the benefits of the Zone diet in the treatment of diabetes dates back to the distant 1998 [39], but since then numerous studies have appeared in the international scientific literature which have shown the superiority of the composition of the Zone diet in reducing the values of Glycemia (blood sugar) [40],[41],[42],[43].

In 2005, the *Joslin Diabetes Harvard Medical Research Center School* proposed its new nutritional guidelines for the treatment of obesity and diabetes; these guidelines were essentially identical to the rules of the Zone.

Studies conducted by *Joslin Diabetes Research Center* following those guidelines confirmed the efficacy of the Zone in reducing risk factors for diabetes [44].

Therefore, those who still persist in saying that the Zone diet is not recommended for diabetics should be told to challenge it to the Harvard University scholars.

THE ZONE IN PRACTICE.

In addition to being effective, a food style must also be feasible, and the Zone is feasible in every situation.

It is only necessary to fill one third of the plate with lean proteins (of animal origin, in this case better or fish, or of vegetable origin such as those derived from soy and lupine) filling the other two thirds of the plate with abundant vegetables and then adding a portion of fruit (i.e. colored carbohydrates).

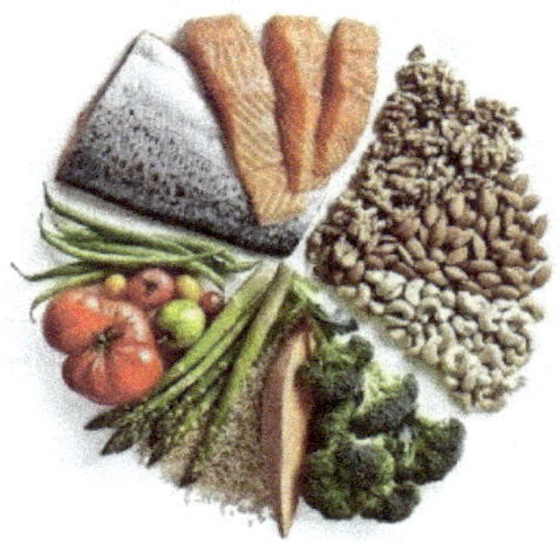

A good combination

A small amount of heart-healthy monounsaturated fat (olive oil) is added to the vegetables.

You can balance the plate as described in the previous sentence using your hand as a measure by eye, getting about 40 percent of your calories from carbohydrates, 30 percent from protein, and 30 percent from fat.

A recent study by the University of Stanford has shown that the Zone diet provides a greater quantity of micronutrients (vitamins, mineral salts, antioxidants) than any other diet [45].

Undoubtedly there are many theories on nutrition, but the Zone is the one that over the years has continued to give the best concrete results both with diabetes and with many other pathologies.

SUPPLEMENTS TO HELP LOWER BLOOD SUGAR

Scientists are testing many different supplements to determine if they help lower blood sugar.

Personally, I remain convinced that nutrition and physical activity remain the pillars against type II diabetes, but since they are still natural products, I think it is useful to illustrate them below, since they could benefit people with prediabetes or diabetes, in particular type 2.

1. CINNAMON

Cinnamon supplements are made with whole cinnamon powder or an extract.

Many studies [46],[47] suggest that it helps lower blood sugar and improves diabetes control.

When people with prediabetes -- meaning a fasting blood sugar of 100-125 mg/dL -- took 250 mg of cinnamon extract before breakfast and dinner for three months, they experienced an 8.4 percent decrease in blood sugar at fasting compared to those taking a placebo [48].

In another three-months study, people with type 2 diabetes who took 120 or 360 mg of cinnamon extract before breakfast saw an 11% or 14% decrease in fasting blood sugar, respectively, compared with those taking a placebo [49].

Additionally, their glycosylated hemoglobin -- a three-month average of blood sugar levels -- decreased by 0.67 percent or 0.92 percent, respectively.

All participants took the same diabetes medication during the study.

How it works: Cinnamon may help the body's cells respond better to insulin. In turn, this allows sugar to enter cells, lowering blood sugar [50].

Intake: The recommended dose of cinnamon extract is 250 mg twice a day before meals.

For a regular cinnamon supplement (not extracted), 500 mg twice daily may be best [51],[52].

Precautions: The common variety of cinnamon Cassia contains more coumarin, a compound that can damage the liver in high amounts. Ceylon cinnamon, [53] on the other hand, is low in coumarin.

2. AMERICAN GINSENG

American ginseng, a variety grown primarily in North

America, has been shown to reduce postprandial blood sugar by approximately 20% in healthy individuals and those with type II diabetes [54].

Additionally, when people with type II diabetes took 1 gram of American ginseng 40 minutes before breakfast, lunch, and dinner for two months while maintaining regular treatment, fasting blood sugar decreased 10% compared with placebo.

How it works: American ginseng can improve the response of cells and increase the body's insulin secretion [55],[56].

Intake: Take 1 gram up to two hours before each main meal: taking it before may cause your blood sugar to drop too low.

Daily doses greater than 3 grams do not appear to offer additional benefits [57].

Precautions: Ginseng may decrease the effectiveness of warfarin , a blood thinner, so avoid this combination.

It can also stimulate the immune system, which could interfere with immunosuppressant drugs [58].

3. PROBIOTICS

Damage to gut bacteria, such as with taking antibiotics, is associated with an increased risk of several diseases, including diabetes [59].

Probiotic supplements, which contain beneficial bacteria or other microbes, offer numerous health benefits and may improve the body's handling of carbohydrates [60].

In a review of seven studies of people with type II diabetes, those who took probiotics for at least two months had a 16 mg/dL decrease in fasting blood glucose and a 0.53% decrease in A1C compared with those treated with placebo [61].

People who took probiotics containing more than one species of bacteria had an even greater decrease in fasting blood sugar of 35 mg/dL [62].

How it works: Animal studies suggest that probiotics can lower blood sugar by reducing inflammation and preventing the destruction of insulin-producing pancreatic cells. Many other mechanisms could also be involved [63],[64].

Intake: Try a probiotic with more than one beneficial species, such as a combination of L. acidophilus , B. bifidum , and L. rhamnosus .

It is not known whether there is an ideal mix of microbes for diabetes [65].

Precautions: Probiotics are unlikely to cause harm, but in some rare circumstances they could lead to serious infections in people with significantly compromised immune systems [66].

4. ALOE VERA

Aloe vera can also help those looking to lower their blood sugar. It may help reduce fasting blood glucose and A1C in people with prediabetes or type II diabetes [67].

In a review of nine studies of people with type II diabetes, aloe supplementation for 4-14 weeks reduced fasting blood glucose by 46.6 mg/dL and A1C by 1.05% [68].

People who had fasting blood sugar above 200 mg/dl before taking aloe experienced even stronger benefits.

How it works: Studies in mice indicate that aloe can stimulate insulin production in pancreatic cells, but this has not been confirmed.

Several other mechanisms may be involved [69].

Intake: The best dose and form is unknown. Common doses tested in studies include 1,000 mg per day in capsule form or 2 tablespoons (30 mL) per day of aloe juice in divided doses [70].

Precautions: Aloe can interact with several medications, so consult your doctor before using it.

It should never be taken with the heart medicine digoxin.

5. BERBERINE

Berberine is not a specific herb, but rather a bitter-tasting compound taken from the roots and stems of certain plants, including goldenseal and phellodendron [71].

A review of 27 studies of people with type II diabetes found that taking berberine in combination with dietary and lifestyle changes reduced fasting blood glucose by 15.5 mg/dl and A1C by 0. .71% compared with dietary and lifestyle changes alone or with a placebo [72].

The review also found that berberine supplements taken alongside diabetes medications helped lower blood sugar more than medications alone.

How it works: Berberine can improve insulin sensitivity and improve the absorption of sugar from the blood into the muscles, which helps lower blood sugar [73].

Intake: A typical dose is 300-500 mg taken 2-3 times a day with main meals.

Precautions: Berberine can cause digestive disorders, such as constipation, diarrhea or gas, which can be improved with a lower dose (300 mg). Berberine can interact with several medications, so consult your doctor before taking this supplement [74].

6. VITAMIN D

We have previously discussed the importance of vitamin D in type II diabetes [75]. In one study, 72% of participants with type II diabetes were vitamin D deficient at study entry [76].

After two months of taking a 4,500 IU supplement of vitamin D daily, both fasting blood glucose and glycosylated hemoglobin improved.

In fact, 48 percent of participants had glycosylated hemoglobin that showed good blood sugar control, compared to just 32 percent before the study.

How it works: Vitamin D can improve the function of insulin-producing pancreatic cells and increase the body's responsiveness to insulin [77],[78].

Intake: Ask your doctor for a vitamin D blood test to determine the best dose for you.

The active form is D3, or cholecalciferol , so look for this name on supplement bottles [79].

Precautions: Vitamin D can trigger mild to moderate reactions with different types of medications, so ask your doctor or pharmacist for advice.

7. GYMNEMA

Gymnema sylvestre is an herb used as a treatment for diabetes in the Ayurvedic tradition of India.

The Hindu name of the plant - *gurmar* - means *"sugar destroyer"*.

In one study, people with type II diabetes who took 400 mg of gymnema leaf extract daily for 18 to 20 months experienced a 29 percent decrease in fasting blood sugar. Glycosylated hemoglobin decreased from 11.9% at study entry to 8.48% [80].

Further research suggests that this herb may help reduce fasting blood sugar and glycosylated hemoglobin in type 1 (insulin-dependent) diabetes and may reduce cravings for sweets by suppressing the sweet taste sensation in the mouth [81].

How it works: Gymnema silvestre can reduce the absorption of sugar in the intestines and help cells absorb sugar from the blood.

Because of its impact on type 1 diabetes, it is suspected that Gymnema silvestre may in some way help the insulin-producing cells in the pancreas.

Intake: the recommended dose is 200 mg of Gymnema leaf extract twice a day with meals. **Precautions:** Gymnema silvestre can increase the blood sugar effects of insulin, so use it only with the guidance of a doctor if you take insulin injections.

It can also affect the blood levels of some drugs and one case of liver injury has been reported [82].

8. MAGNESIUM

Low blood levels of magnesium have been observed in 25-38% of people with type II diabetes and are more common in those who do not have their blood sugar under control [83].

In a systematic review, eight of 12 studies indicated that giving magnesium supplements for 6-24 weeks to healthy people or people with type II diabetes or prediabetes helped reduce fasting blood sugar levels, compared with a placebo.

Furthermore, each 50 mg increase in magnesium intake produced a 3% decrease in fasting blood glucose in those who entered the studies with low blood magnesium levels [84].

How it works: Magnesium is involved in normal insulin secretion and the action of insulin in body tissues.

Intake: The doses given to people with diabetes are usually 250-350 mg per day.

Be sure to take magnesium with a meal to enhance absorption [85].

Precautions: Avoid magnesium oxide, which can increase the risk of diarrhea.

Magnesium supplements can interact with several

medications, such as some diuretics and antibiotics, so consult your doctor or pharmacist before taking them [86].

Magnesium supplements are available online.

9. ALPHA - LIPOIC ACID

Alpha-lipoic acid , or ALA, is a vitamin-like compound and a potent antioxidant produced in the liver and found in certain foods, such as spinach, broccoli, and red meat [87].

When people with type II diabetes took 300, 600, 900 or 1,200 mg of ALA along with their usual diabetes treatment for six months, fasting blood glucose and A1C decreased more as the dose increased.

How it works: ALA can improve insulin sensitivity and the uptake of sugar from the blood into cells, although it may take a few months to experience these effects.

It may also protect against oxidative damage caused by high blood sugar levels.

Intake: Doses are usually 600-1,200 mg per day, taken in divided doses before meals.

Precautions: ALA may interfere with treatments for hyperthyroidism or hypothyroidism.

Avoid very large doses of ALA if you are deficient in vitamin B1 (thiamin) or struggle with alcoholism [88],[89].

10. CHROMIUM

Chromium deficiency reduces the body's ability to use carbohydrates, converted into sugar, for energy and increases insulin requirements [90].

In one review of 25 studies, chromium supplements reduced A1C by approximately 0.6% in people with type II diabetes, and the average fasting blood glucose decrease was approximately 21 mg/dl, compared with a placebo [91].

A small amount of evidence suggests that chromium may also help lower blood sugar in people with type 1 diabetes [92].

How it works: Chromium may enhance the effects of insulin or support the activity of insulin-producing pancreatic cells.

Intake: A typical dose is 200 mcg per day, but doses up to 1,000 mcg per day have been tested in people with diabetes and may be more effective.

The *chromium picolinate* form is probably better absorbed [93].

Precautions: Some medications, such as antacids and others prescribed for heartburn, can decrease chromium absorption.

PHYSICAL ACTIVITY

Another fundamental aspect for reducing blood sugar is physical activity. In addition to the benefits on all fronts, it suffices to say that physical activity also improves depression as well as boosting our immune defences, preventing tumors and cardiovascular disorders.

Given that the muscles are the first users of glucose, it is clear that physical activity has the primary result of lowering blood sugar.

Below are two tables illustrating the energy requirements of a 70 kg man for one hour both in sporting activities and in other activities of common life.

Good movement !

Activity	Calories	Activity	Calories
Aerobics	440	Gymnastics	180
Mountain climbing	600	Golf	240
Baseball	300	Judo	720
Basket	480	Karate	720
Billiards	50	Swimming	600
Bowling	250	Water polo	720
Boxe	850	Volleyball	540
Hunting	200	Fishing	120
Soccer	500	Ping pong	180
Canoe	350	Fencing	600
Cycling	660	Squash	840
Running	900	Archery	280
Equitation	400	Windsurf	200

The values do not include the requirement for basal metabolic rate

Sew	30
Moderate exercise bike	425
General gymnastics	215
Go shopping	95
Doing massages	215
Shopping	60
Gardening	215
Watching television	10
Drive a car	75
Wash the car	80
Working at the computer	18
Working at the desk	10
Stroll	180
Give the vacuum cleaner	250
Clean the house	110
Split the wood	30
Shoveling snow	350-1.100
Shoveling snow	355
Sweep	215
Standing	18
Press	40-90
Play an instrument	60
Tapis Roulant	440
Trekking	565
Yoga	140
Digging	290-600

The values do not include the requirement for basal metabolic rate

WHO AM I

I am a Nutritionist and a Psychologist.

I have worked for over 30 years in various clinics in Tuscany -Italy, in the nutrition sector, also with people with eating disorders.

I was a contract professor at the Faculty of Medicine of the University of Pisa and in others. I continue to consult online through my website. **www.dietazonaonline.com**

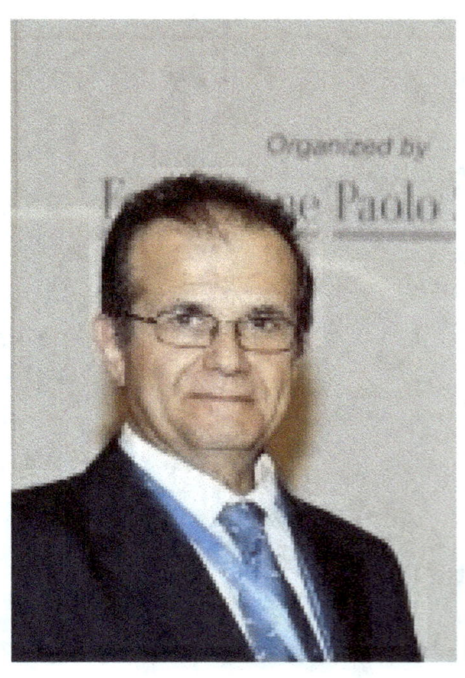

To find out more about me you can go to my curriculum https://dietazonaonline.com/curriculum-vitae-dott-buracchi

If you want you can write to
g.buracchi@gmail.com

If you are interested in my other books on nutrition, natural health, psychology and novels find me on Amazon https://www.amazon.it/s?k=gabriele+buracchi

MY ENGLISH BOOKS ON AMAZON

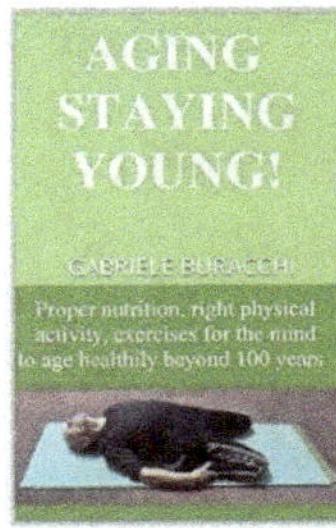

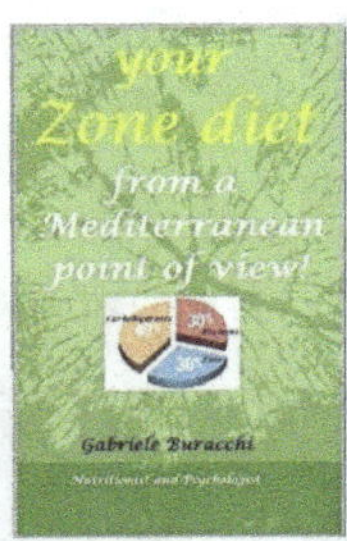

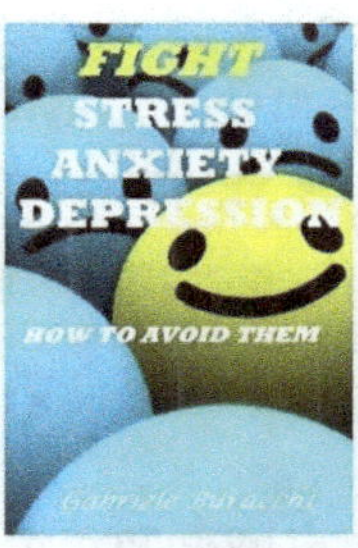

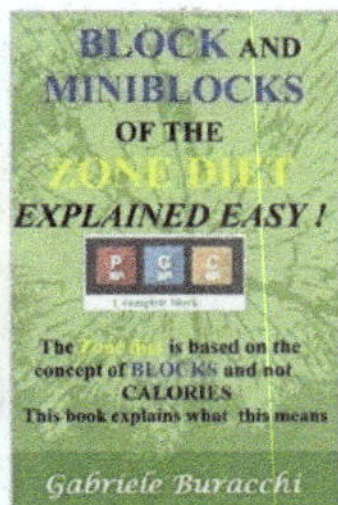

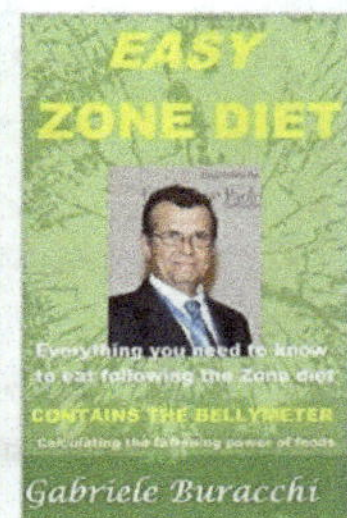

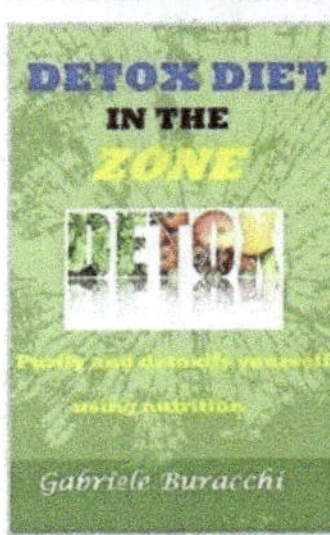

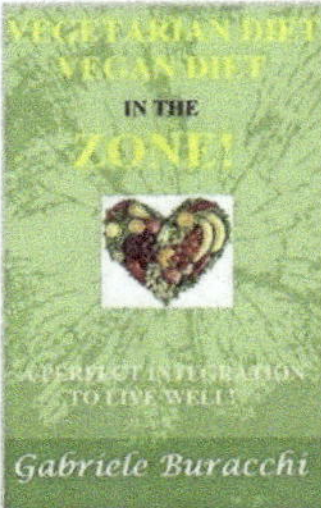

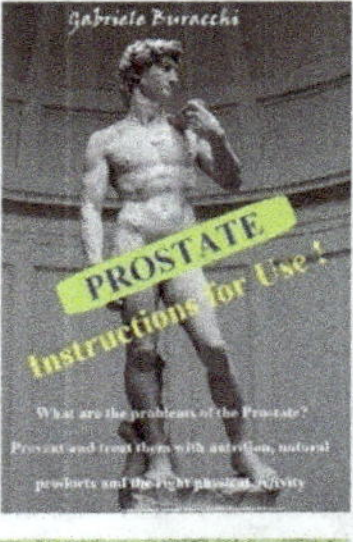

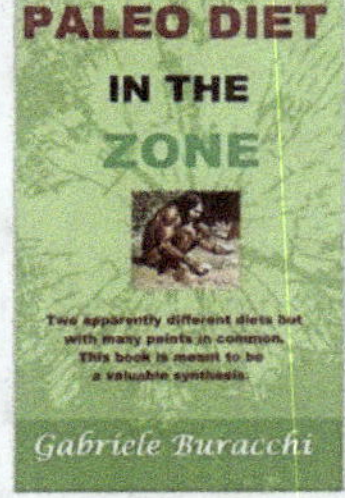

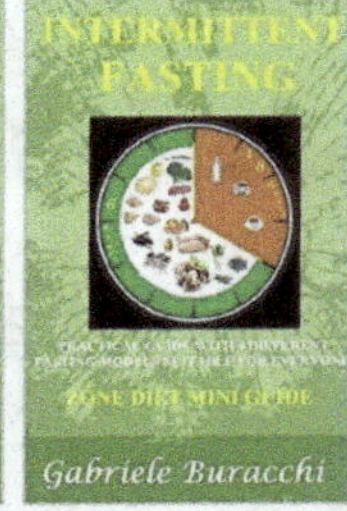

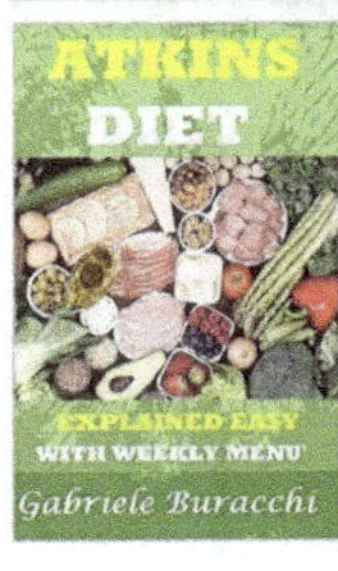

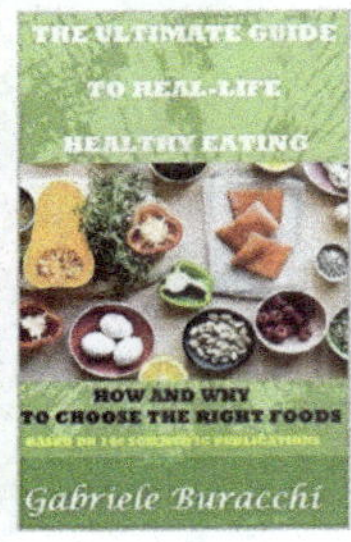

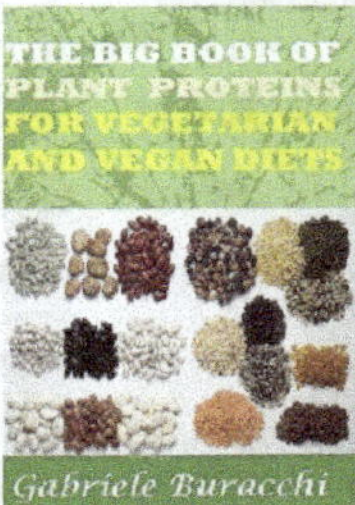

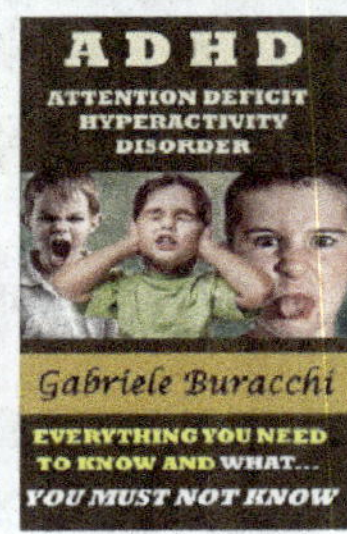

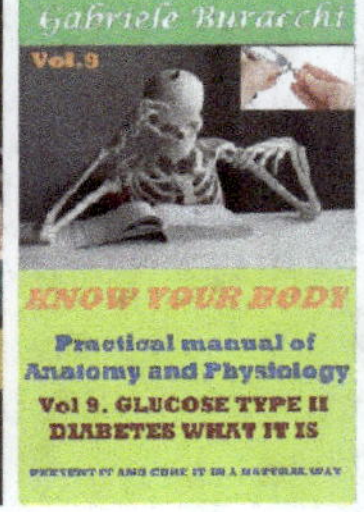

BIBLIOGRAPHY

[1] [1] https://www.diabetes.co.uk/symptoms/polyuria.html

[2] https://www.nei.nih.gov/learn-about-eye-health/eye-conditions-and-diseases/diabetic-retinopathy

[3] https://www.aoa.org/healthy-eyes/eye-and-vision-conditions/diabetic-retinopathy?sso=y

[4] https://journals.plos.org/plosone/article?id=10.1371/journal.pone.0165652

[5] https://www.nature.com/articles/s41467-020-18276-0

[6] https://apic.org/monthly_alerts/diabetes-infections-and-you/

[7] https://www.ncbi.nlm.nih.gov/pmc/articles/PMC5296448/

[8] https://www.niddk.nih.gov/health-information/diabetes/overview/preventing-problems/sexual-bladder-problems

[9] https://onlinelibrary.wiley.com/doi/10.1111/j.2047-2927.2013.00083.x

[10] https://www.diabetes.co.uk/low-testosterone-and-diabetes.html

[11] https://www.ncbi.nlm.nih.gov/pmc/articles/PMC4346284/

[12] https://www.niddk.nih.gov/health-information/diabetes/overview/preventing-problems/sexual-bladder-problems

[13] https://www.cdc.gov/diabetes/basics/pcos.html

[14] https://www.niddk.nih.gov/health-information/diabetes/overview/preventing-type-2-diabetes

[15] https://www.health.ny.gov/diseases/conditions/diabetes/prediabetes/

[16] https://www.niddk.nih.gov/about-niddk/research-areas/diabetes/diabetes-prevention-program-dpp

[17] https://diabetes.org/diabetes/genetics-diabetes

[18] https://pubmed.ncbi.nlm.nih.gov/23700533/

[19] https://www.diabetes.co.uk/waist-measurement-diabetes-risk.html

[20] https://www.niddk.nih.gov/health-information/diabetes/overview/what-is-diabetes/prediabetes-insulin-resistance

[21] https://diabetesjournals.org/spectrum/article/24/4/234/31830/Drug-Induced-Glucose-Alterations-Part-2-Drug

[22] https://www.ncbi.nlm.nih.gov/pmc/articles/PMC4420570/

[23] Fresh fruit consumption in relation to incident diabetes and diabetic vascular complications: A 7-y prospective study of 0.5 million Chinese adults - PMC (nih.gov)

[24] https://www.acog.org/womens-health/faqs/gestational-diabetes

[25]https://academic.oup.com/ejendo/article-abstract/181/3/287/6654148? redirectedFrom=fulltext

[26]https://pubmed.ncbi.nlm.nih.gov/20215450/

[27] https://pubmed.ncbi.nlm.nih.gov/27002059/

[28] https://www.ncbi.nlm.nih.gov/pmc/articles/PMC3942667/

[29]https://reader.elsevier.com/reader/sd/pii/S0002916522004944? token=4A5073D7A113D24342AD8298EA24AA921D3618232C3706DE28D95 4DF659103612A70C91520D7FA2E39A3A2EE5F780E6C&originRegion=us- east-1&originCreation=20230301085519

[30] Skov AR, Toubro S, Ronn B, Holm L, and Astrup A. "Randomized trial on protein vs carbohydrate in ad libitum fat reduced diet for the treatment of obesity." Int J Obes Relat Metab Disord 23: 528-536 (1999).

[31] Layman DK, Boileau RA, Erickson DJ, Painter JE, Shiue H, Sather C, and Christou DD. "A reduced ratio of dietary carbohydrate to protein improves body composition and blood lipid profiles during weight loss in adult women." J Nutr 133: 411-417 (2003)

[32] Fontani G, Corradeschi F, Felici A, Alfatti F, Bugarini R, Fiaschi AI, Cerretani D, Montorfano G, Rizzo AM, and Berra B. "Blood profiles, body fat and mood state in healthy subjects on different diets supplemented with omega-3 polyunsaturated fatty acids." Eur J Clin Invest 35: 499-507 (2005)

[33] Layman DK, Evans EM, Erickson D, Seyler J, Weber J, Bagshaw D, Griel A, Psota T, and Kris-Etherton P. "A moderate-protein diet produces sustained weight loss and long-term changes in body composition and blood lipids in obese adults." J Nutr 139: 514-521 (2009

[34] Ebbeling CB, Leidig MM, Feldman HA, Lovesky MM, and Ludwig DS. "Effects of a low-glycemic-load vs low-fat diet in obese young adults: a randomized trial." JAMA 297: 2092-2102 (2007)

[35] Pittas AG, Das SK, Hajduk CL, Golden J, Saltzman E, Stark PC, Greenberg AS, and Roberts SB. "A low-glycemic-load diet facilitates greater weight loss in overweight adults with high insulin secretion but not in overweight adults with low insulin secretion in the CALERIE Trial." Diabetes Care 28: 2939-2941 (2005)

[36] Larsen TM, Dalskov SM, van Baak M, Jebb SA, Papadaki A, Pfeiffer AF, Martinez JA, Handjieva-Darlenska T, Kunesova M, Pihlsgard M, Stender S, Holst C, Saris WH, and Astrup A. "Diets with high or low protein content and glycemic

index for weight-loss maintenance." N Engl J Med 363: 2102-2113 (2010)

[37] Ludwig DS, Majzoub JA, Al-Zahrani A, Dallal GE, Blanco I, Roberts SB, Agus MS, Swain JF, Larson CL, and Eckert EA. "Dietary high-glycemic-index foods, overeating, and obesity." Pediatrics 103: E26 (1999)

[38] Agus MS, Swain JF, Larson CL, Eckert EA, and Ludwig DS. "Dietary composition and physiologic adaptations to energy restriction." Am J Clin Nutr 71: 901-907 (2000)

[39] Markovic TP, Campbell LV, Balasubramanian S, Jenkins AB, Fleury AC, Simons LA, and Chisholm DJ. "Beneficial effect on average lipid levels from energy restriction and fat loss in obese individuals with or without type 2 diabetes." Diabetes Care 21: 695-700 (1998)

[40] Layman DK, Shiue H, Sather C, Erickson DJ, and Baum J. "Increased dietary protein modifies glucose and insulin homeostasis in adult women during weight loss." J Nutr 133: 405-410 (2003)

[41] Gannon MC, Nuttall FQ, Saeed A, Jordan K, and Hoover H. "An increase in dietary protein improves the blood glucose response in persons with type 2 diabetes." Am J Clin Nutr 78: 734-741 (2003)

[42] Nuttall FQ, Gannon MC, Saeed A, Jordan K, and Hoover H. "The metabolic response of subjects with type 2 diabetes to a high-protein, weight-maintenance diet." J Clin Endocrinol Metab 2003 88: 3577-3583 (2003)

[43] Gannon MC and Nuttall FQ. "Control of blood glucose in type 2 diabetes without weight loss by modification of diet composition." Nutr Metab (Lond) 3: 16 (2006)

[44] Hamdy O and Carver C. "The Why WAIT program: improving clinical outcomes through weight management in type 2 diabetes." Curr Diab Rep 8: 413-420 (2008)

[45] Gardner CD, Kim S, Bersamin A, Dopler-Nelson M, Otten J, Oelrich B, and Cherin R. "Micronutrient quality of weight-loss diets that focus on macronutrients: results from the A TO Z study." Am J Clin Nutr 92: 304-312 (2010)

[46] https://pubmed.ncbi.nlm.nih.gov/30144878/

[47] https://pubmed.ncbi.nlm.nih.gov/22953038/

[48] https://pubmed.ncbi.nlm.nih.gov/18500972/

[49] https://pubmed.ncbi.nlm.nih.gov/22953038/

[50] https://pubmed.ncbi.nlm.nih.gov/26475130/

[51] Investigation of the biological properties of Cinnulin PF in the context of diabetes: mechanistic insights by genome-wide mRNA-Seq analysis - PubMed (nih.gov)

[52] https://pubmed.ncbi.nlm.nih.gov/14633804/

[53] https://pubmed.ncbi.nlm.nih.gov/25905290/

[54]Efficacy and safety of American ginseng (Panax quinquefolius L.) extract on glycemic control and cardiovascular risk factors in individuals with type 2 diabetes: a double-blind, randomized, cross-over clinical trial - PubMed (nih.gov)

[55] https://pubmed.ncbi.nlm.nih.gov/25905290/

[56] https://pubmed.ncbi.nlm.nih.gov/27547829/

[57] https://pubmed.ncbi.nlm.nih.gov/25905290/

[58] https://pubmed.ncbi.nlm.nih.gov/25905290/

[59] https://www.emjreviews.com/diabetes/article/role-of-probiotics-in-diabetes-a-review-of-their-rationale-and-efficacy/

[60] https://pubmed.ncbi.nlm.nih.gov/26987497/

[61] https://pubmed.ncbi.nlm.nih.gov/26987497/

[62] https://pubmed.ncbi.nlm.nih.gov/26987497/

[63] https://www.emjreviews.com/diabetes/article/role-of-probiotics-in-diabetes-a-review-of-their-rationale-and-efficacy/

[64] https://pubmed.ncbi.nlm.nih.gov/26987497/

[65] https://pubmed.ncbi.nlm.nih.gov/26987497/

[66] https://juniperpublishers.com/apbij/pdf/APBIJ.MS.ID.555606.pdf

[67] https://pubmed.ncbi.nlm.nih.gov/25905290/

[68] https://pubmed.ncbi.nlm.nih.gov/27152917/

[69] https://pubmed.ncbi.nlm.nih.gov/27347994/

[70] https://pubmed.ncbi.nlm.nih.gov/23035844/

[71] Meta-analysis of the effect and safety of berberine in the treatment of type 2 diabetes mellitus, hyperlipemia and hypertension - PubMed (nih.gov)

[72] https://pubmed.ncbi.nlm.nih.gov/25498346/

[73] https://pubmed.ncbi.nlm.nih.gov/18442638/

[74] https://pubmed.ncbi.nlm.nih.gov/18397984/

[75] https://pubmed.ncbi.nlm.nih.gov/29672520/

[76] https://pubmed.ncbi.nlm.nih.gov/26391639/

[77] https://pubmed.ncbi.nlm.nih.gov/21715514/

[78] https://pubmed.ncbi.nlm.nih.gov/23674796/

[79] https://ods.od.nih.gov/factsheets/VitaminD-HealthProfessional/

[80] https://pubmed.ncbi.nlm.nih.gov/2259217/

[81] https://pubmed.ncbi.nlm.nih.gov/2259216/

[82] https://pubmed.ncbi.nlm.nih.gov/20856101/

[83] https://pubmed.ncbi.nlm.nih.gov/9589224/

[84] https://pubmed.ncbi.nlm.nih.gov/28526383/

[85] https://pubmed.ncbi.nlm.nih.gov/11756061/

[86] https://ods.od.nih.gov/factsheets/Magnesium-HealthProfessional/

[87] https://pubmed.ncbi.nlm.nih.gov/22374556/

[88] https://pubmed.ncbi.nlm.nih.gov/1815532/

[89] https://pubmed.ncbi.nlm.nih.gov/7649494/

[90] https://ods.od.nih.gov/factsheets/Chromium-HealthProfessional/

[91] https://pubmed.ncbi.nlm.nih.gov/24635480/

[92] https://pubmed.ncbi.nlm.nih.gov/9451374/

[93] [93] https://pubmed.ncbi.nlm.nih.gov/9356027/

www.ingramcontent.com/pod-product-compliance
Lightning Source LLC
Chambersburg PA
CBHW070752250726
48662CB00004B/1771